CHEMICAL-FREE KIDS